FOR THE LOVE OF SPA AND WELLNESS

(A CONSUMER'S GUIDE TO SPA, BEAUTY AND

WELLNESS)

BY

EUNICE NONAN IBUS ESTIPONA

&

TED T TAVERNIER

ISBN: 978-1493652945

DEDICATION

Dedicated to all those whose

passion is in spas,

massage therapy

and wellness

If you are serious about getting started in this industry,

then read her book:

"Spa, Massage Therapy, and Wellness Resource Book

and Career Guide" by Eunice Estipona

www.SpaBusinessResource.com

FOR THE LOVE OF SPA AND WELLNESS

(A CONSUMER'S GUIDE TO SPA, BEAUTY AND WELLNESS)

TABLE OF CONTENTS

Chapter I

What You Should Know

It was one of those days that I wanted to receive a massage, and in that afternoon, our regular "Hilot" just dropped by our house out of nowhere. I will refer to her as "Manang Lucing" (definitely not her real name). No one had recommended Manang Lucing to us. In fact, she just comes whenever she feels the need to come. She doesn't even have a mobile phone. "Manang Lucing" is in her mid-60's, petite and thin and always wearing skirts because it is her belief that women should always wear skirts. She has long hair which more often than not is either clipped or in a ponytail, but nothing notably fancy about her. She has been our "hilot" for more than a decade now. So, I have high praises for her services and recommend this "hilot".

By the way, let me educate my non-Filipino readers. Hilot means two things, the art of massage from techniques learned from tradition and the person performing the massage (noun). It doesn't really jive with modern science and medicine, but it has been in our culture for many centuries.

Our session usually starts with me lying face down on our massage bed (Yes, I do have a massage/facial bed and three massage chairs at home- does it show you how addicted I am to massage? Hehe…) working first on my thighs or my back. After thirty minutes or so, I was half asleep. Yes, it was pure bliss!

Okay, so back to the beginning. This particular day in August while I was having my "Hilot" session, my Tatay (or Tay , as we fondly call our father) was having a vacation at home instead of the country. My father was listening and half observing while reading the paper in the other room. He saw how relaxed I had become and decided that he also wanted to have a "Hilot" session. He had been complaining of backaches several days earlier, so I told him to have a session too. After more than an hour, I stood up and called my father to get ready. Meanwhile, I gave Manang Lucing a snack before she worked on my dad.

When she was ready, I said "Your turn, Tay " He was pretty excited because he wanted to get rid of his aches. As usual,

Manang Lucing started with a short prayer and I could sense that the first three minutes were a pure bliss for my father until Manang Lucing started to work on his back. His back has a lot of lamig or sometimes massage therapists call them nodules or knots.

After those two minutes, you could hear my father say from time to time "Arayyy" (Ouch!) but Manang Lucing was oblivious to what she was hearing and she kept on working on his back with vigor and enthusiasm. Sometimes, it's an "aray" with a whispering "a" and sometimes it's "Arrayyyy" with a capital "A".

My poor father, what has he done to deserve this? It was as if my father was being tortured. I giggled a bit knowing that even when I massaged him gently he would still say "Aray". For the entire hour or so, he was saying "Aray" sometimes loud and sometimes in whispers. It's a good thing that our next door neighbors are not as close together as they would have wondered what was happening.

Then after more than an hour or so of great service for me and excruciating pain for my father- he was reluctant to pay Manang Lucing for nearly killing him. What the heck, he was relieved afterwards and was advised not to take a shower or bath for the next 24 hours.

Hilots believed that "knots" came from open pores and since the body is warm from the massage your pores are open. Then if you take a bath your pores will close with engulfed air within the skin and that becomes a "knot" in the long run.

Hilot

So here I am a spa operations and management consultant- getting a great massage from an uneducated, high school graduate "hilot"- not because of her education or the techniques but because of the relief she brings to my shoulder pains. Even though I know that she is un-licensed and un-certified, I still keep on availing myself of her services because she meets my needs as a client. I did not care about diplomas, licenses and degrees as I wanted someone who could deliver results. This is unconventional. I am not saying that diplomas, licenses and degrees do not count, but as a client I would rather experience results more than anything else.

The spa, massage therapy, beauty and wellness is also filled with technical details and professional regulations, but I am not going to bore you with that. I hope I can make everything as clear and as simple as possible. So I already defined hilot. We have two schools of thought regarding the use of hilot: one as a traditional healing therapy and the other for relaxation. For example, a "hilot" practitioner in one locality may practice different techniques than a hilot practitioner in another locality. We have to accept that traditionally, hilot is practiced through folk medicine and thus cannot be placed in a box. Some principles can be explained by Science and some we just have to accept that even in Hilot, some questions in this world can never be answered by a finite mind. It doesn't mean that it is not effective. For example, we can't totally explain the existence of air or love but it doesn't necessarily mean that it is non-existent. There maybe a few practices that cannot be explained by Science, but that doesn't mean it's not effective.

The "Hilot" principle is different from every region and although they have similarities they also have differences. As I said earlier Manghihilots or Hilots are Filipino traditional healers based in communities who deliver health services. During the Spaniard and American era this was largely ignored and suppressed. So, why are there no "hilots" that are multi-millionaires? It is because the cost of a consultation is free or voluntary. Our old manghihilots before believe that it lessens the "Hilot's" healing powers. In the olden days, one does not go to a hilot when they don't feel anything is wrong with them. Therefore as doctors have specializations, hilots also have their own specialty. Common categories of hilots: arbolarios (folk doctors), herbalist (manganganga or arbolaryo or herbolaryo), obstetrician (partera, nagpapa anak or comadrona). As we have evolved into modern Science, we depended less and less with Hilots.

So what should you expect during a hilot session? To name a few, Hilots may perform body scanning on or above the client's back. Some of hilot's diagnostic methodologies include: pulse reading, thermal diagnosis (hot and cold), phrenology/ physiognomy, urine, skin and perspiration analysis. Some hilot practitioners apply warm strips of herbs or banana leaves before and after a massage. Most hilot practitioners use "coconut lana" or oil from coconut or use virgin coconut oil to lace these herbs which are then applied on the client's skin. They said that these leaves are naturally ionized and possess astringent and cleansing properties. Sometimes a client will also be asked to bathe ("banyos") in a warm or lukewarm solution of guava leaves for 15 to 20 minutes before a hilot session. The guava leaves, especially the shoots, are boiled and while still hot placed in a container, normally a pail of water and then bathed by the client warm or lukewarm. There is also the practice of "oslob" or "suob", this is the steam inhalation of dried aromatic herbs usually" Bayabas (guava), sambong, lemon grass in a basin for 5 to 10 minutes. Sometimes an arbolaryo will ask you to chew young guava leaves and swallow it to help in coagulation. If one has a fresh wound like during circumcision, the guava leaves can be masticated then applied externally to minimize bleeding. Herbs normally used during hilot are sambong (English: Elumea or Ngaicamphor; Scientific name: *Blumea balsamifera*), lagundi (English: Five-leaved Chaste tree; Scientific name: *Vitex negundo L.*), Ilang- ilang (English: Ylang-ylang; Scientific name:

Cananga odorata), peppermint (Scientific name: Mentha peperita) and ginger (Tagalog: luya; Scientific name: *Zingiber officinale*).

Manghihilots or Hilots (the noun version) believe that everything is labeled hot or cold thus, the term "may lamig ka". On a massage therapist's point of view, these are called "knots" or "nodules" which needs to be kneaded. These accumulate when the body is exposed to too much warmth (therefore pores open) then an exposure to coldness in temperature or may result from abrupt changes in temperature thus the open pores close abruptly with trapped air inside. In Science, any strenuous activity that makes us tired and sweaty open our pores especially during warm climate then when we expose ourselves in an air-conditioned room, the result of which is a disruption of the natural internal balance. So "Hilots" warn parents to keep infants dry because "malalamigan" especially the bumbunan (or the anterior fontanelles). If you have a sprain, you go to a "hilot" if you need to be kneaded go to a massage therapist.

There are certain situations and conditions that are contraindications in hilot but not contraindicated by massage and there are also certain situations that are contraindicated in massage but not in hilot. Let's differentiate some methodologies of massage and hilot. In massage, generally, sprains are contraindicated but not in hilot. In massage (as thought by Western countries) you can take a bath, but in hilot you are never encouraged to take a bath after a hilot. You can have a massage even when you have a menstrual period and this is definitely avoided in hilot. Because hilots say that during menstruation, our body is prone to hematoma and pain tolerance is lower than usual.

There is another Filipino Indigenous Therapy called "Kolkolis" or "Dagdagay", a foot massage originating from Mt. Province, Sagada, Tadian. Sometimes pine sticks are applied like drum sticks on the feet.

Services for hilot and other indigenous therapies are generally a bit higher than other whole body massage due to the preparation and training involved. Fees range anywhere from P500 (approximately $10) to as much as P5,000 (approximately $115) depending on the establishment you go to. When it comes to prices and rates, there are high-end spas, middle of the road and low end ones. Whereas a one hour whole body massage of Swedish, Shiatsu or Thai only costs P1,000 and as low as P200 in some establishments. Some are worth the money you pay for and others are just a total waste of money. So if possible, you need to read the reviews and testimonials online. But the best advice is to have someone you trust and/ or a professional recommend an establishment to go to.

Spa and Massage Therapy

Spas on the other hand are originally places for bathing, healing and relaxation. Today there are establishments offering these rituals of bathing and they have gone far beyond the original concept. The modern spas are establishments offering varied products and services from relaxation, health maintenance, fitness activities, nutrition counseling, facial therapies, body treatments, massage and bodywork and a whole lot more. Spas exist in all shapes and sizes, you can find them in resorts (that is why they are called resort spas), hotel spas (within a hotel facility), airport spas (located inside airports), and even inside malls- or what we sometimes call day spas or mall spas. There are different kinds of spas differentiated by the services they offer or their location. There is no one definition of a spa as the word is used in other industries like a dental spa, car spa, pet spa, etc. All of which address a need that the market is willing to pay for.

According to the Philippine Department of Tourism, a spa is an establishment that has a holistic approach to health and wellness, rest and relaxation that aims to treat the body, mind and spirit by integrating a range of professionally administered health, wellness, fitness and beauty, water treatment and services. With this definition, you can see that there are establishments that don't fit under the definition of a spa. A salon (or parlor as it is commonly called) would not become a spa salon or spa-lon just by simply adding a foot spa service or a foot spa machine. A doctor's office that performs diamond peel services does not automatically qualify as a medical spa (or medi-spa), but that they are business establishments offering a spa service. The establishment has to have a combination of several typical spa services to be called a spa.

Common among which are:

Body Treatments: Different types of wraps like: herbal wraps, mud wraps, seaweed wraps, aromatherapy wrap, etc.

Massage and Bodywork: Swedish, Shiatsu, Thai, Reflexology, Acupressure, etc.

Facial Therapies: European, anti-aging, deep cleansing, whitening, oxygen, diamond peel, etc.

Hydrotherapy: sauna, steam bath, Vichy/Swiss shower, hydrotherapy bath, etc.

Fitness: Pilates, yoga, Aerobics, Tai-chi, hiking, etc.

Salon services: Paraffin dip, haircut, styling, manicure, pedicure, foot spa, hand spa, etc.

Lifestyle classes: nutrition counseling, healthy cooking, vegetarianism, organic food preparation, raw food preparation, sleep enhancement programs, music therapy, etc.

Medical treatments: Botox, diamond peel, micro-dermabrasion, acupuncture, etc.

Not All Services are the same

Although there are many benefits of a massage, there are also things that a consumer should be aware of. There are many medical conditions in which massage is not appropriate. The body is being compromised by these conditions and massage may worsen the situation. If you are not sure, check with your doctor before having a massage. It's better to be safe than sorry. Below are some tips, precautions and contraindications of massage:

Ø   Edema or pagmamanas- Areas of swelling, edema or pagmamanas. This is due to the fact that there might be an underlying systemic cause to this edema and as massage therapists, we do not want to aggravate the situation. It is better if the client consults first with a physician.

Ø   Fever- Whole body massage is not allowed with people who have high fever. If you have headaches and a slight fever, a light gentle massage on the forehead to just relieve the pain can be given, but whole body massage is not recommended. The reason is that, you will be subjecting your body to working overtime in order to counteract any toxin effects and at the same time excrete them. We do not want to overwork the body as it needs rest when you have a fever. At the same time, the fever might be caused by an infection. Until that infection is being addressed, I would like to advise you to refrain from a whole body massage.

Ø Bruising or hematoma or pasa- It is better not to touch the bruised area.

Ø Broken Bones- Go to a doctor instead but in some cases, those with sprains are being healed by a "hilot". As I said earlier, I do not want to be dogmatic. There are some medical conditions that are a no-no for massage but okay with "hilot". It's up to your discretion. Consult first with an orthopedic doctor or your family physician.

Ø Various heart conditions like high blood pressure- If you have high blood pressure and not on medication, then this is a no-no. Especially if your blood pressure is really high or more than 120/90.

Ø Varicose veins- Should not be given too much

pressure during a massage.

Ø   Never massage directly on infected skin- example, where there are warts, boils or where there is inflammation (pamamaga), unexplained lumps (hindi maipaliwanag na bukol), bruises and cuts.

Ø   If pregnant- Although there is what we call pregnancy, maternal or prenatal massage, it is best avoided during the first three months of pregnancy when the risk of miscarriage is highest.

Ø   If you have a period or menstruation- In Western thought, you can have a massage even if you have menstruation but, in our age old traditional Hilot, this is a no-no. They say that this is sometimes the reason why your period suddenly stops after the massage session. We do not want that because a monthly period is considered dirt that the body should excrete.

Ø   Do not eat heavily right before a massage- wait at least two to four hours after meals before having a massage.

Ø   It is advisable not to drink alcoholic beverages, smoke, take a bath or expose yourself to cold right after a massage as this will alter the temperature of your body and shock your systems. Thus, will not be good for the over all well-being. As much as possible, hot beverages like "ginger tea or salabat" or warm water is advisable rather than drink "iced tea". Why is it important if it's hot or warm? Because after a massage, your body has been exposed to heat and the last thing you want to do is to expose yourself immediately to cold temperature. So give it time to adjust. Our old people call them "lamig" (or what massage therapists refer to as nodules or knots). There could be some truth in it, as sudden change of temperature is also not good for the body.

Ø   Be open to your massage therapist- If you feel any discomfort say so. If the speed of movement, pressure or technique needs to be changed, then say so and feel free to give feedback. When asked about any health-related information, give your therapist accurate health information and do not withhold anything that is worthy of mentioning.

A professional massage therapist should be able to ask you about your medical history (amongst other things): If you have any allergies, a history of high blood pressure, what area would you like to focus on, etc. With the information/data that you have given them, they will also be able to assess the right type of massage/pressure for you or if they should refer you to another health care provider.

Ø   Frequency/Duration- Please note that massage has its greatest benefits over time. So, the more regular your massage is, the better you will feel in due time and the more quickly the body will respond to the therapy. For general preventive health maintenance, a 60-minute massage every two weeks or at least once every fifteen days is the ideal frequency. In cases of specific problems or dysfunction, more often is recommended (once every four days at the most), until an appropriate outcome is achieved.

Legal Issues

When it comes to legalities what do you need to know? In the Philippines, PD 856 of Chapter XIII Sec. 9.1.1 states that no person is authorized to practice massage in the Philippines without holding a valid certificate of registration for masseur issued by the Committee of Examiners for Massage Therapists and approved by the Secretary of Health. This means, if we are to be technical and dogmatic, any person is not allowed to perform massage without a license. Most specifically if it is your source of income. Not unless you are under the direct supervision of a Licensed Massage Therapist.

But it doesn't mean that if you are not licensed then you are not talented in your craft. There are a lot of massage therapists out there who are great and skilled in what they do even though they are not licensed. I think the best solution for this is self-regulation. The massage therapist should assess the client well and adopt certain techniques in massage that would help the client and not harm them in any way. The practice of any profession including massage is done with a clear conscience Period! As a client, assess the professionalism of your therapist and go with your gut instinct. Go to credible spas and massage clinics who make good on their promises and have a high regard for quality. Do not always go for the cheapest one around. Sometimes, it pays to ask your friends and family members whom they recommend.

If you have the money and are qualified, then by all means get a license. It will add to your credentials. Generally, a massage is non-invasive. So, no need to worry as massage has been used for centuries and centuries.

There are more than 400++ types of massage and we will only discuss the common forms. The massage therapies differ in pressure, techniques, and history or origin.

Pressure - light, moderate, or medium and hard (which is what Filipinos love)

Techniques- The feet are used (like Ashiatsu), the clients are lifted and stretched (like Thai), warm stones are applied on clients body (like Stone massage) etc.

History- Depending on the country of origin. Reflexology came from China with roots in Egypt, Shiatsu came from Japan and Thai massage came from Singapore …no just kidding. Obviously, it came from Thailand! (Thai Yoga massage originated in India).

There are also differences in the types of lubricant that massage therapists use. Sometimes, they use oil, cream, gel, lotion, powder or none at all. So it all depends on the type (or sometimes referred to as modality) of massage and the massage therapist or client's preference. Whichever one uses, it should have a beneficial effect to the body.

Client preparation- You are naked, half-naked, or fully-clothed depending on the treatments, but draped. Generally, only (as applicable) shorts with underwear are worn unless otherwise indicated.

Time or Duration- Massage therapies generally run an hour or two.

There are no regulations (yet) regarding the practice of spa therapies in the Philippines. Beauty Therapies on the other hand and Wellness Hilot is being regulated by the Technology and Skills Development Authority (TESDA).

How to Differentiate the Types of Massage

It is equally important for consumers and massage enthusiasts to know if you are getting the right kind of massage for you specific needs. The following below are the most common:

Acupressure- This type of massage technique is for certain areas only, it is not designed as a whole body massage or application (otherwise you might mistake this as a Shiatsu) and it can be applied with our without lubrication, medium to hard pressure. The massage therapist may or may not use wooden sticks for massage, but generally they use their fingers and thumbs.

Aromatherapy Massage or Aromassage- This is being incorporated into many massage modalities where the massage therapist uses authentic (not synthetic) organic oils. These are essential oils blended with a carrier oil, commonly called an Aromatherapy massage. So a Swedish massage can be an Aromatherapy massage if the oils used are true essential oils and not synthetic ones. If these oils are plant-based it can also be considered Phytotherapy incorporated into massage. But how can you be sure if it's really organic and natural? Buy from reliable, credible sources and FYI, these oils are not cheap. Beware of imitations and cheap oils like mineral or baby oils used claiming to be Aromatherapy.

Chair Massage or On-Site Chair Massage- This type can be performed sitting upright on a stool, a low backed chair or a professional massage chair. This can be done in just five, ten, fifteen minutes to nearly an hour. Most commonly done for 20-30 minutes where the focus is on the back and shoulder area, nape and head. Normally the therapist uses cream as a lubricant and the client is fully clothed. This can be incorporated with acupressure, hand reflexology or Indian head massage. If its Indian head massage, then it may include the back, shoulders, arms/hands, nape/neck, head/scalp and face.

Deep Tissue- These techniques include cross-fiber friction, stretching, and trigger-point release. Just as the name implies, deep, meaning do not expect gentle pressure here. This is not a massage for relaxation but to ease aching muscles and knots. It is basically used to enhance sports performance and recuperation. It's an effective component of any training program. Often it is integrated with other massage methods. It may or may not be a whole body massage as the therapist may focus on certain areas that are being specifically used in sports. Like the groin and legs if the client is a runner. It also involves some form of stretching and range of motion techniques. Duration is normally one hour to two hours. The difference between Deep Tissue and Sports massage is that it incorporates deep tissue techniques before or after a major sports event to bring blood to critical parts of the body and loosen muscles. While this is done, athletes visualize their best performance, supporting muscle memory that helps maximize their training and effort.

Geriatric Massage- This is the opposite of infant or pediatric massage which has some form of gentle techniques specific to ease joint pains and other chronological symptoms of aging.

Hilot- There are a lot of conceptions (and misconceptions) regarding Filipino traditional hilot which has already been discussed in great detail in the previous section. Historically, hilot is considered a healing modality. An herbal application with coconut oil is common. Sometimes, sampaguita and ylang-ylang essential oils are blended with the coconut oil. Some other techniques or practices which can be added to the experience include pulse reading, skin analysis, thermal diagnosis, banyos, suob or oslob (steam inhalation of aromatic herbs) amongst others. It can run from an hour to more than two hours. Hilot is not only relaxing but a healing therapy in itself. I suggest every Filipino to try this out so we will be able to appreciate our culture and heritage in this modality.

Hot Stone Massage- These are warm smooth stones applied either before or during the massage. It can also be integrated into some types of massage. The therapist typically uses Swedish massage techniques with the stones placed on your spine, palms of your hands and in between your toes, etc. It runs from an hour to two hours. This is more expensive than a typical massage because of the required preparation needed and the duration. These stones may also be used to massage certain areas of your body. A variation of this is the herbal ball massage, common in Thailand where the herbal ball contains specific herbs, heated and applied on certain areas, especially the back and shoulders to relieve aches and pains. If you have persistent back pain, I recommend this type of massage (only if there is no underlying cause, just muscular in origin). It may seem that it's a wise idea to buy mechanically polished stones but there are a lot of factors in choosing the right stone. Mechanically polished stones are NOT recommended because mechanical polishing seals up the stone's surface. It's preferable to get them from nature where they've been polished to perfection by streams and oceans.

Infant/ Baby or Pediatric Massage- Just as the name implies, it's a gentle massage done on babies or children. This is a great way for babies and children to get started on a life-long enjoyment of massage therapy. It provides stimulation of the nervous system, touch and supports the parent-child bonding.

Manual Lymph Drainage or Lymphatic Drainage Massage- It is sometimes referred to as slimming massage or anti-cellulite massage because of its pumping and suction techniques to improve the flow of lymph by using light and rhythmic strokes. A gentle form of massage, duration is one hour to two hours depending on the spa, massage clinic or wellness center.

Pregnancy, Maternal, Maternity or Prenatal Massage- This is another variation of Swedish massage but focusing on relieving the discomforts of pregnancy.

Reflexology- This is a popular and ancient form of Chinese Bodywork. If we are to be technical about this type or massage, authentic reflexology only focuses on the feet, hands and ears, not the whole body. So technically speaking, there is no such thing as whole body reflexology. Today, reflexology is incorporated into many massage modalities and spa services like foot and hand spa services. This is a medium to deep compression massage which uses thumb and finger pressure (but the therapist may use instruments and lubricants to aid in the process) as there are specific points in the hands, feet and ears that correspond to the nerve endings of a particular organ or muscle. It is said that if your reflexologist comes to a tender spot on one of those extremities, pay heed to the organ or system to which it may be connected because it might signify health concerns in your body.

Relaxation, Classical, European or Swedish Massage- It is generally a gentle to medium pressure massage that generally uses lubricants and a system of gliding strokes, kneading and friction techniques in the direction of the blood flow toward the heart. This is the most common form of massage and typically runs for one hour only. It is my recommended massage for first timers. This is a bit of a misnomer here because the name Swedish Massage, was neither invented by a Swede nor developed in Sweden, despite massage therapy books that say so. It was a Dutch practitioner Johan George Mexger (1838-1909) who gets credit for adopting the French names that define the basic massage strokes- effleurage, petrissage, friction and tapotement - and systematizing them into what would most accurately be called Classic massage. In any case, this technique is the foundation for most massage therapy practice today.

Shiatsu- is a Japanese form of whole body, medium to hard pressure, fully clothed massage, similar to a Thai massage. It is done on a floor mat using the therapist's finger, knuckles or thumb and may run from one to two hours long using no oil. Techniques may include: pounding, stretching, rocking and manipulation techniques. Pressure may be applied by the use of forearms, elbows, palms, feet and knees. Meanwhile, Ashiatsu uses the bare feet of the therapist while the therapist holds on to an oriental bar hanging from the ceiling. Watsu (Water-Shiatsu) is Shiatsu done in the water. So you see, massage evolves in time with new techniques being invented.

Signature Massage- The techniques and style are created by the owners and are specific only to that spa. The massage may be a combination of three or more massage modalities running from thirty minutes, to an hour or two hours long.

Thai Massage or Nuad Bo Ram- This is a more rigorous type as compared with other forms of massage because Thai massage employs a series of range of motion stretches as well as combines active and passive movements of joints. Therefore this is not recommended for those who have difficulty in stretching or who has bone problems. It is generally performed on a comfortable floor mat to allow maximum mobility that would allow the therapist to utilize their body weight. The client is fully clothed and no lubricant is required. Western style requires the client to undress for oils to be applied on the body and the massage is most often performed on a massage table. Typically this runs from one to two hours long.

Although massage lost some of its value and prestige with the unsavory image created by "massage parlors", this image is slowly fading as awareness of the value and therapeutic properties of massage grows. Thanks to the proliferation of day spas around the globe, Massage Therapy is no longer viewed as a sexual service but a way to rejuvenate mind and body. So, professional massage therapists may terminate a session because of any illicit or sexually suggestive remarks or advances from the client. Although not a substitute for medical care, massage can reduce or eliminate the need for medication and surgery. Massage today is not only used for humans but pets and animals as well. A variety of massage techniques are now being incorporated into different programs and alternative/complementary therapies including osteopathy, chiropathy, etc. Massage Therapy has now gained popularity with not only well-off individuals, but the common people as well, thus making wellness for everyone and not only for those who have the money.

Massage therapy has evolved with time and you can combine techniques, adjust the pressure or make your own steps. There will be new discoveries everyday so keep an open mind. We do not have to be dogmatic or too strict on steps and procedures. For as long as the result is a better, rejuvenated client, then I do not think there is anything wrong with that. There are also numerous forms of massage styles that I have not mentioned. In short, there is a lot to learn out there and you can enjoy the many variations of massage therapies.

Facial Therapy

A facial is either a light or deep cleansing of the face by various means including; steam, exfoliation, extractions (manually or by machine), the application of creams, lotions, masks, peels, toning, and of course a facial massage. It cleanses, exfoliates, tones and nourishes the skin to promote clear, well-hydrated skin. A facial will improve the appearance of your skin and relax you at the same time. It is the second most popular spa service after massage.

Professionally, a facial is given by a licensed Esthetician with special training in skin care. Most dermatology clinics today also offer clinical facials.

Ideally, get a facial every four to six weeks because that's how long it takes the skin to regenerate. Try to have a facial at least four times a year, if you have a clear complexion and are following proper skin care. You may need it more frequently if you are trying to clear up a case of acne, especially at the beginning. Hint: For normal skin, use your age to determine how many days apart to schedule your next facial. Example, if you are twenty years old you need to go for a facial every twenty days. But nobody follows it because it's easier to remember once a month or twice a month for regularity purposes.

European facials cleanse, steam, extract, exfoliate, massage, mask, tone and moisturize the whole face, neck, décolleté and sometimes the bust area. Variations on the classic European facial include the "mini-facial" (cleansing without extractions) and specialty facials. Add vitamin C, and you have an "age defense" or "anti-aging" facial. It's called an "oxygen facial" when a mist of pure oxygen is part of the treatment, and a "collagen facial" when special collagen sheets or plain collagen are placed on the skin. An "acne" facial will pay special attention to extractions and focusing on pimples, acne and drying them up.

Contraindications in a facial treatment:

1. Skin disorder- such as acne vulgaris (unless medical approval has been sought and given)

2. Skin disease- impetigo

3. Bruising in the area

4. Hemorrhage

5. Surgical Operations

6. Fracture

7. Furuncle (boil)

8. Inflammation/Swelling of the skin- or too sensitive skin

9. Scar Tissue

10. Eye disorders

11. First trimester of pregnancy

12. Hypersensitivity (allergy) to skin products

A range of different products are available in the market for facial therapy, some examples are:

1. Cleansers

2. Face wash

3. Face scrubs

4. Exfoliants

5. Toners

6. Moisturizers

7. Face mask

8. Oxygenating preparations

9. Ampoules

Aesthetics-   Defined as the study or theory of beauty. It was the youngest branch to be given its own name which was first used in 1700's. Since 1800's, writers have been developing aesthetics into a more independent field of study.

Note: Before a facial treatment, a skin analysis is generally performed to see what type of facial best suits your skin. If you are a returning client, the Esthetician will want to see if there are improvements on your skin.

CHAPTER II

Beauty Addiction

The reason why there is a burgeoning of facial centers, anti-aging clinics and esthetics businesses in the Philippines (and even worldwide) is that believe it or not, deep in the recesses of the human mind, we are humans who do not like to get old, have wrinkles and die. We stop counting when our age is not in the numbers of the calendar. We resort to cow poison so our wrinkles don't show. We even contour everything from head to toe, hate fats, flabs and wrinkles, even defying gravity on our cheeks and bellies. Lagnat na lagnat tayo sa mga Botox (Botox fever), We have anti-aging mania like Justin Beaver's mania, anti-wrinkles, anti-cellulite, etc. Anything that defies gravity on our facial muscles and body contours, oh we love these! We somehow have the notion that the more beautiful we are on the outside, then the more acceptable we are to society. Thus, people will like and believe in us.

Listed below are some of the most popular procedures that require a board certified plastic or cosmetic surgeon. Do not gamble your life and your body. Select a surgeon you can trust. Someone who is professionally trained and experienced in all plastic surgery procedures, including breast, body, face and reconstruction. Someone who operates only in accredited medical facilities, adheres to a strict code of ethics, fulfills continuing medical education requirements, including standards and patient safety, and has your best interest at heart.

As always, there will be a preliminary consultation to determine if you are a good candidate for any procedure and to go over some pre-surgery instructions from your board certified plastic surgeon. They want to be certain that you are an ideal candidate for the procedure or just a patient who should seek less invasive alternative treatments like body contouring, thermo-shaping or just plain old diet and exercise. Therefore, a consultation with your plastic surgeon is very important. Common procedures include the following:

Face lifts – or technically called Rhytidectomy is a very detailed surgery that requires a board certified face lift surgeon or plastic surgeon, not just a dermatologist. A face lift is like waging war against gravitational pull on the face. A face lift is performed to remove sagging skin, reduce excess skin, reduce the appearance of wrinkles and creases on the face. A face lift that is well done will not be obvious and will have minimal scarring. The trick here is to make it more natural. So, to be sure seek the advice of specialty doctors in well known hospitals and ask for their assistance. They might give you some other alternatives besides a surgical procedure like a face lift. There are also anti-aging gadgets that might temporarily help delay the time at which a facelift becomes appropriate and complement the results of surgery. Take note, a facelift does not change your fundamental appearance and cannot stop the aging process.

Botox- is actually a toxin from the bacteria Clostridium botulinum that causes muscular paralysis. Botox is a temporary treatment for frown lines and brow furrows where the toxin is injected into muscles in between the eyebrows (glabellar lines) and/ or forehead in people 18 to 65 years of age for a short period of time (temporary). Botox essentially paralyzes the muscles and stops them from contracting. So even if you laugh or frown, your face won't show the emotion. Botox injection is usually performed with some local anesthesia or a numbing cream. Depending on the extent of treatment, the procedure can take anywhere from a few minutes to 20 minutes. Results are visible within one week after treatment and remain for a minimum of three months. You can resume normal activities immediately, but your doctor may advise you to stay out of the sun. Again, it's best to consult with your dermatologist or go to a reputable medical spa.

Tummy Tuck – or Abdominoplasty is another surgical procedure performed by a board certified plastic surgeon and is often performed with general anesthesia. The tummy tuck surgery takes about two to five hours. Tummy tucks maybe an option if you have loose sagging skin on your abdominal muscles that cannot be removed no matter how many sit-ups and exercises you do. Men and women alike can enjoy the benefits of a tummy tuck.

Breast or bust augmentation- or Augmentation mammaplasty surgery involves using breast implants to fulfill your desire for fuller breasts (breast enlargement) or to restore breast volume lost after weight reduction or pregnancy (breast enhancement).

Butt or Buttock enhancement – Some women want to enhance the size of their rear end and having a beautiful, rounded and firmly shaped "J Lo" buttocks has always been and probably always will be considered the most attractive and desirable attribute of a woman. As a result many of our plastic surgeons specialize in buttock implants or buttocks shaping and contouring.

Dermabrasion- It is most often used to reduce or remove scars left by accidents or a previous surgery or to smooth fine facial wrinkles. Dermaplaning is commonly used to treat deep acne scars. Both dermabrasion and dermaplaning can be performed on small areas of skin or on the entire face. They can be used alone, or in conjunction with other procedures such as a facelift, scar removal or revision, or chemical peel. There is also what they call Micro-dermabrasion or micro-resurfacing which is a non-invasive procedure where only a tiny layer of the skin is scratched to remove fine lines and dead skin cells. Micro-dermabrasion can be performed by a skin care professional or Esthetician. It is being marketed as an alternative to the costlier and invasive procedures such as chemical peels, plastic surgery and Botox. Many different products and treatments are used in conjunction with this method, including medical procedures, salon treatments, creams, and scrubs that you apply at home. It's usually done to the face, chest, neck, arms or hands. The most common example is the diamond peel where an electrical machine sucks out the debris of your face while scratching the skin's surface. This however, is not advisable for real sensitive skin and those whose work is prone to sun exposure.

There are more beauty therapies out there including facials, body wraps: slimming wraps, herbal wraps, retail products like anti-aging, whitening, nutritional supplements, etc. that are all geared toward fixing our outward appearance. If you are white, you darken your skin (by tanning, tanning salons, solariums and tanning lotions, etc). If you are brown or black you whiten you skin (by bleaching, whitening pills like glutathione, etc.). If you are in your teens, you want to look like a grown-up so you wear make-up and wear adult dresses. If you are in your mid-thirties and above, then you want to look young. So you dress up like teenagers and wear light make up. If you have long hair, you cut them. If you have short hair, you make them long or wear hair extensions. Isn't it ironic?

However, there was a man in history for whom appearance did not matter. Actually, if you are to look at his old photos, it was the least of his assets, ang maging pogi (being handsome). This person was Abraham Lincoln who knew he was not a handsome man. Edwin Stanton, a political opponent of Abraham Lincoln, often called Lincoln a "gorilla" even in public debates. Lincoln never let his appearance bother him even if other people used it to insult him. No political figure has been insulted for his looks more than Abraham Lincoln. But he never took a grudge against Stanton even when he became president and appointed Edwin Stanton as his Secretary of War. Maybe if we were Abraham Lincoln we would never appoint a political opponent especially those who ridicule us and say "you are ugly". Even Lincoln's friends objected to his decision because Stanton was known for ridiculing Lincoln. When asked why he was choosing Stanton, Lincoln replied "because I know he is the best man for the job". This is one of the many reasons why Stanton became a Republican and apparently changed his opinion of Lincoln. At Lincoln's death Stanton remarked, "Now he belongs to the ages," and lamented, "There lies the most perfect ruler of men the world has ever seen."

(Above: Abraham Lincoln Courtesy of www.visitingdc.com)

Stanton vigorously pursued the apprehension and prosecution of the conspirators involved in Lincoln's assassination. This is one of the many reasons why Abraham Lincoln turned out to be one of the greatest Presidents, if not the greatest President of the United States. He recognized a person's worth no matter how that person has hurt him. He didn't rely solely on physical appearances.

Again, when it comes to physical appearances, who would have thought that a black African American with a middle Eastern sounding name would be elected as the 44th President of the United States? His full name is Barack Hussein Obama. He recalled, "That my father looked nothing like the people around me — that he was black as pitch, my mother white as milk".

Incidentally, the inauguration of President Barack Obama as the forty-fourth President, and Joe Biden as Vice President, took place on January 20, 2009. The theme of the inauguration was "A New Birth of Freedom," commemorating the 200th anniversary of the birth of Abraham Lincoln.

In my own humanity, I was once labeled as "the little brown director". My color has been a stigma for me since I was in the Elementary grades where my classmates would tease me and call me a "niger", "black" "uling" and "ita". I somehow thought that my skin color is inferior and bad. So when I became an adult, I strived to have a more fair skin color. Thereby, taking all necessary whitening, bleaching agents, tablets, going to expensive procedures just to make my skin lighter, whiter, etc. because I was not proud of my skin color. Well of course, those procedures did succeed to some extent. I am no longer as dark as before, but after all those things, I realized it's not the color of my skin that really matters in the long run. It's the color of one's heart. Beauty is indeed in the eyes of the beholder. Thankfully, I overcame that vanity, little by little.

Another person whom I met that did not judge people by appearance was Dr. Noah McKay, Author of the Book, "Wellness at Warpspeed". To those who have met him in person, I know that you recall only his gratitude, love, and everlasting hope for humanity and healthcare. I and thousands of people out there will always be thankful to God for the short but wonderful experience with him. I am still hopeful for the future of medicine and healthcare worldwide. He passed away February 13, 2009, at the age of 52 and just like most Filipinos who are delighted by food, he also loved food. Yes, I can still recall when I introduced him to our amiable Dean who was also my former Professor, Dr. Nini Festin Lim, who told him that I am one of the brightest in class (to my surprise!). Dr. Noah replied, "yes, she is, I know and I never doubted that". His message of love and gratitude inspired thousands of people at seminars and public appearances everywhere. He encouraged us to integrate love and gratitude back into our family, our relationships our careers, and institutions. He dreamed of a day when we teach an educational curriculum based on love, compassion and non-violence at our schools and colleges. Our future and the future of our planet will depend on it. Hats off to you Dr. Noah! You are a visionary. You believed so much in the capacity of human nature and what we can do to make this world a better place to live in. You will be missed. We thank you, your family and wife Kim, for sharing your wisdom.

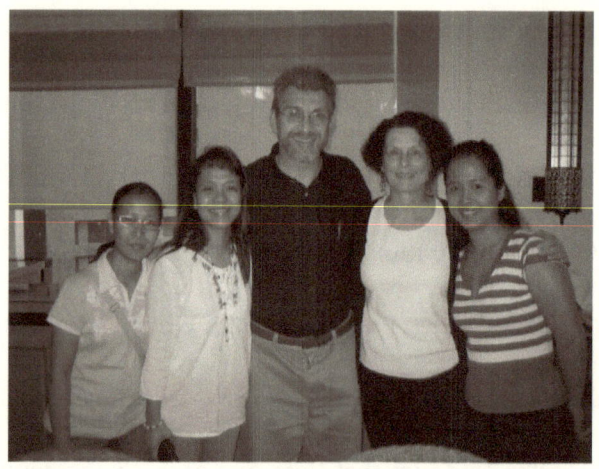

(Above: L to Rt: Cathy Benavidez, Eunice Estipona, Dr. Noah McKay, Kathy Tomlan et al)

I remember a story about a soldier who was physically handicapped and finally coming home after the Vietnam War. He called his parents in San Francisco, California and told them he

48

was coming home, but never seemed to have the courage to tell them about his condition of losing an arm and a leg. Instead he told his parents that "I am bringing home a friend with me". "Sure" his parents replied. "He was hurt pretty bad in the fighting and stepped on a land mine losing an arm and a leg, and has nowhere to go". Their son requested that his friend live with them. The parents told their son "I'm sorry to hear that son, maybe we can help him find a place to live." But their son was unwavering in his decision, "I want him to live with us". "Son," the father replied, "You don't know what you're asking. Someone with a handicap will be such a terrible burden to us. We all have our own lives to live and we can't let something like this interfere with our daily lives. I think you should just come home and forget about this friend of yours. He will find a way to live on his own." The son hung up and the parents heard nothing more from him. A few days later, the parents received a phone call from the police station and told them that their son died after falling from a building. The police believed it was suicide. The grief-stricken parents traveled all the way to the city morgue to identify the body of their son only to find out, to their shock that their son, had only one arm and one leg.

The parents in this story are common to most of us. We find it easy to accept those who are good looking, rich, beautiful or fun to be with, but we do not like people who are fat, physically challenged, who inconvenience us or those who are unlike our skin color or race. We sometimes judge a person by appearance.

We do not realize that these people are hurting too and that somehow, there is this unwritten law inside our head that says, "you must keep your emotions inside you and do not bother other people with your weakness and hurts". We project an image of ageless beauty but our hearts struggle with pain. Now is the time for us to respond to our friend's hurts, our neighbor's cry and become sensitive. Are you willing to open up a home in your heart where they can be accepted no matter what? Do not believe in myths that it's better not to have wrinkles. Aging is inevitable but aging with wisdom gained from life's experiences and lessons are commendable. Therefore, we age gracefully. We do not pick or choose what part of our loved ones life we can accept and not accept. As I recall the movie "Connie and Carla" with one of my favorite actors David Duchovny, they said, "That is why God placed those laugh lines, let your eyes crinkle, your skin wrinkle…these lines show that we have lived!" and "when your love partner doesn't love you when you look like a map tell him to hit the road….!" But they have a good point! When we place too much emphasis on the outside appearance, then that is where imbalance happens.

For those people who had been ridiculed, teased and given the cold treatment because you seem to be just ordinary, you are not! You are original, the one and only in the sight of God. Cultivate your talents, find true friends who will not judge you for how and what you look like. God created each of us through His likeness and image. So don't be afraid to shine. God created you to be unique and there is no one else like you on this planet. Wherever you are…..Shine!

CHAPTER III

Who Do You Go For What?

Please consult your doctor in any current condition you have or if current symptoms persist prior to receiving treatment. As in anything, like your skin's condition, your health is attained through years and years of taking good care of it. Avoid disappointment through quick fixes.

When you have acute back and shoulder pain, go to a spa and ask if they provide massage therapy. You can ask the massage therapist or technician to concentrate on the areas which need to be kneaded or are painful. One of their primary responsibilities is to provide custom tailored massage therapies for clients. Also, to suggest the progression for massage therapy services.

While most would agree that beauty begins on the inside, beauty therapists or their counterpart offer services designed to alleviate skin disorders or generally help improve and beautify the skin. Estheticians, Facial Therapists, Skin Care Technicians, and Beauty Therapists are qualified to carry out a wide range of treatments to the face and body. The wide range of beauty therapy treatments does not only include skin care for the face like cleansing, toning and soothing preparations done for the face, but also for the body. It may include eyebrow and eyelash treatments, body waxing treatments, depilation or epilation, eyelash tinting, etc. Aside from manual treatments, beauty therapists often use electrotherapy and other machines and equipment to be able to treat skin and body conditions. They are normally working inside spas, medical spas or clinics and may assist the dermatologist or plastic surgeon.

Nail technicians focus more on nail services mainly manicures and pedicures.

Beauticians focus more on make-up and salon services like: hair cutting, styling, dyeing, hot oil, hair relax, hair straightening, etc.

Spa therapists are the people knowledgeable in all aspects of body heat and wet treatments like scrubs, exfoliations, wraps, masks, hydrotherapy, floatation, steam, sauna, hot tub and cold plunge. Some spa therapists may focus on other treatments like health and fitness. They will work with a team of other specialists such as nutritionists to be able to create a treatment plan for individual clients.

If you want to learn Yoga, Pilates, Tai-chi and other exercise regimens then go to wellness trainers, fitness instructors or teachers employed in full scale spas, wellness centers or fitness centers.

Generally, for your hair services go to a salon where your stylist can create a custom amazing look just for you. They can suggest amazing color with depth, dimension, shine and style. They have different hair treatments from coloring, cutting and finishing. Services in a salon include nails and hair and most often than not, they also offer hand and foot spa services. Some salons offer massage and other facial services, but inquire first to be sure.

A day spa comes in all forms and sizes. A full scale day spa offers a range of water-based beauty and fitness treatments from facials to massage, to weight loss counseling. It is similar to a beauty salon in that it is only visited for the duration of the treatment and there is no overnight accommodation. Day spas can be stand-alone, freestanding, or connected to health clubs, hotels, and department stores. Most mall spas nowadays focus more on massage and facial therapies. In comparison, a destination spa, health resort or retreat spa is where you get all of the benefits of a full scale day spa plus accommodations. A destination spa facility's primary purpose is to provide individual services for spa-goers to develop healthy habits. All guests come for a full-immersion experience that is focused on health and well-being. Guests stay typically over a seven-day period. These facilities provide a comprehensive program that include massage and spa services, physical fitness activities, wellness education, healthy cuisine and special interest programming like healthy cuisine, educational classes and seminars. They have similar services of a beauty salon or day spa, but guests reside and participate in the program at a destination spa instead of just visiting for a treatment or pure vacation. They offer structured, personalized programs amid a community of like-minded people. Some destination spas are in exotic locations or in spa villages and towns. An example is the Farm at San Benito in Batangas , Philippines .

CHAPTER IV

Who is Your Best Friend?

Conversation can sometimes be a point of controversy because some clients like to talk during a session while others like silence. I believe it's up to the client to dictate this aspect. The practitioner does not inhibit speaking nor does she/he initiate conversation if the client is silent. If you want to tactfully make certain that your therapist is not overly conversational, then it is appropriate to state something like, "You will find that I am not very talkative. I just would like to completely rest during this time." He/she will get the point. At some time, your practitioner might communicate aspects of the massage or the facial, so please don't take this as trying to make conversation.

Why do people confide in therapists and beauty professionals instead of their spouses or significant other? If they are that significant then how come they get the news last? These people go to the spa and they complain about their spouses and when they come home they complain about the spa. Why? Because the circumstances that you complain about are situations that you can change- but you have chosen not to. You won't complain about air, gravity, the sun or the moon… You won't hear anyone complain about it because you can't do anything about it. We don't complain about things we have no power over.

It's easier to complain than to do something about it. It takes a lot of courage to tell your spouse or significant other that you are not happy with the relationship. It takes courage to ask for a change of behavior from people and we don't know how they would take it. It might be uncomfortable, difficult, alarming to the other party or confusing. You run the risk of failure, confrontation, a broken relationship or just being plain wrong. So to avoid them, you stay put and complain about it. Do not complain to the wrong person who cannot do something about your situation.

When it comes to complaints, we have to learn to make requests and take action that will achieve our outcome. If you find yourself in a situation that you don't like, then you have to decide to make it work or leave. Either way you will get some things changed. As the old adage goes, "Don't just sit there (and complain) do something." It's up to you to change, do, or say something different.

When it comes to personal issues and private lives of clients, it's easy to open up with the ones who really will not be hurt, but will provide an objective analysis of your situation. Remember your beauty therapist is not your Psychiatrist, nor your counselor. But I know in a way, the therapist acts like your junior non-judgmental Psychologist. The therapist and/or beautician is not there to tell you how to live your life. Some topics can be prohibited by law so check with your local jurisdiction on what those off-topics are.

CHAPTER V

Juicy Secrets Consumers Need to Know

For first timers and veterans in the spa, massage and wellness industry, there are a lot of issues and concerns that can be addressed when it comes to Spa Ethics and Etiquette. So, what are the acceptable norms? Even experienced spa-goers can be unclear about customary protocol.

Differences in customs and traditions in one's country also play a role in spa protocol. For example, it is customary to tip 15-20% of the full service price in America. But in Asian countries like Thailand, the Philippines, Hong Kong, Taiwan, etc. it will generally depend on how "gallant" or "generous" a client is. T.I.P.S. is an acronym for "To Insure Prompt Service" or sometimes referred to as gratuity. In the Philippines an acceptable tip depends on the industry, because we also tip waiters, cab drivers, airport helpers, even our laundry ladies, etc. Below is my personal gratuity giving guide for any spa, massage clinic, wellness centers and similar establishments:

No gratuity for terrible service

20 to 50 pesos (approximately $1) is cheap; only for service that is so-so

100 pesos (approximately $2) is fine; for good service

200 pesos (approximately $4) is wonderful; for above standard service

500 pesos (approximately $10) is exemplary; for way above the average service

1,000 pesos and up (approximately $20) is great generosity; for highly commendable service

Of course in other countries, this might sound very minimal as tips are generally 15 to 20% of the service price. If the service price is $50, a client is expected to give $10 minimum. So, then what am I trying to arrive at? My bottom line here is whether you are in the Philippines or anywhere else in the world for that matter, give whatever you are comfortable giving. Give within your means and give out of the abundance of your heart to give. It is not the amount actually, but our attitude about giving.

To get the most out of your therapies and treatments, be on your best behavior, starting at the time you book your appointment. Always consider the role of the receptionist, "the gatekeeper" as you want to start out with a good first impression. If the receptionist or concierge feels like you are a difficult client, then she may actually make a note in the system. This will alert the therapist or stylist of your behavior. You certainly do not want that because if you have an attitude problem, you might get a really mediocre treatment. But on the other hand, if you are able to present a charming and accommodating attitude, then you may find yourself a happy client with free add-ons, extra treatment time, complimentary merienda (snacks) and some other freebies. Be nice, even if it does not guarantee a VIP treatment as it adds to your personality and aura!

Pre-Treatment Preparation

Sometimes we need to be reminded or if new to spa-ing, about pre-treatment planning for your spa visit. If not reminded then you might forget important hygiene activities that are a no-no before your spa-ing time. Some of these examples are; do not cut your nails before a pedicure, or pop a pimple badly before a facial or pluck your eyebrows before shaping or threading- as all of these tend to interfere with what the professionals can do. During or immediately after your period refrain from having a diamond peel, a deep tissue massage or aggressive facial therapies because your pain tolerance is lower during this time and your skin tends to get more sensitive and prone to redness and hematoma (bruising). Avoid shaving the day before an appointment especially if you are having a body scrub or other exfoliation procedures. Scrubs like salt and sugar scrubs are especially irritating on newly shaved skin so notify your therapist. Don't be worried if you have a hairy back as this will not offend your therapist. If you are about to have a salt scrub, a facial extraction or a skin peel then you should not shave because this will heighten your skin's sensitivity to the salt or facial peeling. What I am referring to is shaving the body. If you have a facial, it's generally more acceptable to shave your beard or mustache (it's up to you) several days or a day before your scheduled therapy.

Drink plenty of water before and after a treatment, especially after using the sauna or steam room. Do not overdo it because you might find yourself aching to go several times to the toilet during your massage.

Avoid alcohol the day before your appointment. Refrain from eating or eat only a small amount an hour or two before any treatment.

Draping and Attire

Wear whatever is comfortable. When you arrive at the spa, depending on your treatment or service, they will give you the proper wardrobe to wear. How naked and exposed you'll be depends on the treatments that you will have. When anxious about nudity don't be shy, grab a bathrobe. Ask the receptionist for full details if you're afraid of being completely bare. If you are staying in a hotel or resort, call the spa and find out if it's acceptable to wear your robe from your room to the spa. For clients who have issues regarding their body, it will be hard to imagine yourself getting naked, especially during body scrubs and wraps. Do not worry because the practitioner/ therapists are generally trained to drape you properly and respectfully. Also, if you are having a massage, your therapist is trained in muscle and tissue structure. They will not judge you by your physical appearance. The staff inside the spa sees you as a person and the time you spend with them is a privilege to work with you. If you feel uncomfortable then wear a bathing suit and only take off what you are comfortable with, but don't complain afterwards if there's oil on your luxury linen or underwear. So, if you want to keep your underwear on, then wear the ones that you don't mind getting greasy. Bring your own underwear or you can also ask the spa for a paper thong or disposable underwear which are usually used during scrubs, tanning, bikini wax, etc.

Most spas have changing rooms with lockers, robes and slippers. In a resort, destination, or hotel spa, guests often change in their room and walk to the spa in a robe. But before you go that route, make sure you know where the spa elevator is. It's not cool to end up in the hotel's lobby wearing just a robe.

Being half-naked or nude might be the one aspect that causes guests the most anxiety. Being undressed with someone you have just met may feel awkward, but you do not have to undress completely. Tell your therapist your preference when booking or when you arrive in the treatment room.

A hydrotherapy suite is another area where nudity varies according to one's country. Generally, single-sex sections tend to be bathing suit-optional while coed facilities in Asia and America typically require bathing suits. In some European countries, parts of Japan, Taiwan, and South Korea total nudity is acceptable.

The Issue of Time

In the industry of spa, massage, bodyworks and wellness the issue of punctuality raises some major concerns regarding what is considered punctual. Being punctual may mean 15 minutes before your scheduled massage. It may also mean 30 minutes before your scheduled appointment because you are thinking of using the sauna or hydro-tub first. It's very stressful to think that you have to rush into your facial or massage appointment because you are five minutes late. Do your best to be on time and if possible, early. Spas tend to have a 10-15 minute window when it comes to tardiness- whether it's theirs or the client's. Beyond that, they are definitely due for some compensation.

If you are using the shower, then arrive 20-30 minutes before your treatment time or session. This gives you time to leave the weight of the world behind and adjust to the spa's ambiance. The advantage of being early is that this allows you to prepare for your session. You can relax and enjoy other amenities available within the spa such as the gym, the steam room/sauna or the Turkish bath before the scheduled service begins. So, you tend to be more relaxed and more focused on your session when you are early. Thus get much more from your therapy minutes- valuable minutes which you do not want to waste because you are paying for them. If you are a first-time client, then you might have to fill out some health history intake forms which can again eat up the time. If you have a facial booked for 1 pm and you arrive precisely at 1 pm, the ten minutes you spend finding a locker, undressing and dressing into the spa wardrobe and settling inside the room are all on the clock. If you arrive late, the spa will most likely, charge you for the full session. Sometimes, they can give considerations if there are no appointments or bookings after yours, but do not count on it. Be aware that as professionals/ practitioners, we have already blocked that hour for you and therefore have to turn away other clients who could have benefited from that time.

Budget enough time at the end of your session to have a sip of hot tea, linger in the waiting area, dress up, style your hair, pay the bill, etc. For an hour of service, budget at least 1 hour and 45 minutes out of your day.

When your time is limited or when you are in a rush, it is also a blessing to the staff because they can get some downtime when you leave early. But you must clearly state your situation early on so they can speed up your services or have two people work on you at once.

Generally, the spa can only push your appointment no more than 10 minutes or it's going to cut your treatment time. As stated earlier some great prelude to your session includes the facilities: steam and sauna, tubs and hydrotherapy facilities, etc. If you plan to use all these amenities arrive up to an hour early to take advantage of them.

Bathing, Shower and General Cleanliness and Hygiene

Smelly clients, stinky guests, bad breath, etc. makes treatments unpleasant for the therapist. General guideline dictates taking a bath or showering before your massage or bodywork session.

Shower before entering a whirlpool or a pool.

Sit on a towel when using a sauna or steam room.

Fortunately clients with smelly feet can relax because most spas clean their feet with warm towels and aroma elixirs before any foot procedures e.g. foot spa, reflexology, pedicure, leg massage, etc.

Client Confidentiality and Privacy

To make it easy for everyone, spas always consider privacy. If it concerns other people, do not ask. Records and information are safe in the spa's information vault or database. If the spa needs to release some documents that concern your privacy they will notify you beforehand and have you sign off on a release form.

Unless there is good reason and intention, never place your therapist in an awkward situation like asking about what service or therapies did your aunt, cousin or wife availed of when you were not there. Therapists are professionals and are bound by client confidentiality procedures, just like doctors.

Communication

Generally, people do not have ESP so the principle behind this is 'if you don't ask, (kindly) you don't get". If there is one thing that will make your spa session more enjoyable and beneficial then it is communicating with your therapist. If you are not feeling well, your shoulder is too tender, the stones placed on your back are too hot to bear, you want a more intense massage pressure, you can't hold your need to go to the bathroom, the room is too cold, you need a bolster under your legs, the background music is too loud, or if there is anything that diminishes your enjoyment of, your ability to focus on your session, whatever the issue- by all means, let your therapist know right away! Kindly speak up and communicate with your therapist what your specific expectations are before and/or during the treatments so that you can get back to the business of pampering yourself. Yes, even if you tell the esthetician that the masque or cleanser smells like rotten eggs- break it to them gently. The more directions you give the better. Speak up because one of the biggest mistakes most people make is keeping silent. Communication is the key to getting your needs met.

There is no such thing as painless extractions or a blissful bikini wax as these procedures can be really painful and uncomfortable depending on your pain tolerance. If you experience undue and unbearable stress then ask the therapist to stop. Be polite but direct. Say something like "that area is really sore, can you lighten your pressure a little bit?" or "I would really like more pressure on that particular area" or "I really do not like the smell of that mask, would you mind taking it off?" As the one paying for the session, you have to take the lead and let the therapists know if a particular treatment or something else within the session is making you uncomfortable.

In some spas, it's obvious that staffs are trained to sell retail products, but if you are not interested, a simple "No, thank you" or "Thank you for your suggestions, but I'm happy with just the facial today" should be enough.

Read up on your treatment before going in. Most spas have websites and a spa menu with a description of services that tell exactly what the service entails. You can also call beforehand and ask the receptionist to describe the therapy for you and ask how much? Remember you can always decline a service.

Spas and therapists want your feedback so, if you as a client don't say anything when you are dissatisfied or have any complaints, then you are really doing them a disservice. Because, spas want you to be their client for life, so any dissatisfaction matters. Just be calm (do not rant) and describe exactly what did not meet your expectations and why. By stating your wishes and preferences in a respectful tone, you will not be viewed as demanding or overbearing, as you are actually helping them to make your experience better.

Do not feel like you have to converse once the treatment has begun- go ahead and enjoy it quietly if you wish. But if you want to say something, therapists are happy to oblige. If you found yourself with a chatty therapist, kindly request that you prefer to enjoy your treatment time in silence.

Health Related Questions

Do not neglect to inform the spa of any health related issues you have, like eczema, heart problems, pregnancy, etc. that can affect which treatments you are able to receive.

Don't be afraid to discuss your medical issues so that the therapists will be able to recommend the type of massage, facial, body treatments or any services you should or should not get. If you are allergic to nuts, then say so because they might be using nut oil-based massage oils or scrubs.

Booking, Scheduling Appointments

Almost everyone flocks the spa by evening and on weekends just as everyone wants to have dinner reservations at seven or eight pm. We all want to have the very best massage and the problem could be that the best spa in town is almost always fully booked. Minsan magkakaroon ka ng experience na feeling mo mas maraming naidagdag sa iyong wrinkles kaysa matatanggal na wrinkles sa facial therapy dahil sa hirap magpa-book ng appointment o sa hirap kausap ng nasa kabilang line. (Sometimes as clients, we get more wrinkles trying to land an appointment for that facial than that service was supposed to erase.)

To remedy the situation, be flexible in terms of time of day in order to land a better chance for an appointment. To get those prized time-slots, you have to book in advance and so consider having your spa-ing time at other times of the day. The most quiet timeslots are morning, off-peak season and during weekdays. Plus, hotel and resort spas often offer discounts on off-peak bookings. Let me tell you another secret, the most stressful time to visit the spa is during weekends and holidays or after office hours. I said stressful for both the client and the therapist because you will have a lot of traffic in the hallways, locker areas and waiting rooms. People will be more prone to chatting rather than relaxing. The most peaceful time is during weekday mornings or if you really do not have time in the morning, then Monday and Tuesday evenings tend to be slower than the rest of the week. The evenings on weekends tend to be the busiest. If you decide midway in your session that you would like to get another service or additional therapy time, the spa is not obligated to fit you. But as in any rational business establishment, the spa management might bend over backward to accommodate a client, who wants to spend more time and money at their establishment, especially nice clients. Be sure to book a monthly appointment on your way out because regular clients often get priority.

Noise, Music and Gadgets

If you want to enjoy peace and quiet, the first step is to minimize your own small talk. If it doesn't work and the staff still chatters around you, speak up and emphasize your desire to unwind. If you abruptly say "I don't want to talk", it might make the staff uncomfortable or nervous. But if you would tell him/her something like "I would like to rest my eyes for awhile or I am really looking forward to relaxing during the treatment", they will get the idea.

Buzzing, ringing, vibrating phones, Blackberry and pagers will disrupt your session. Mobile phones and all the other similar devices should be turned off or preferably in your locker, car, at home or endorse it to the concierge. If you cannot make that commitment, postpone the treatment until you are ready.

Which Comes First

Services should always be in the order of body first then face second, and then either feet or hands. But there are a few exceptions which are found below.

Depending on the availability of equipment and staff, and the services to be rendered, some therapies/services can be done simultaneously. A spa pedicure can be done simultaneously with a spa manicure, a facial treatment with a foot spa or a hair service with a spa manicure/pedicure. But if these services cannot be done simultaneously, services should always be in this order; body first then face second and either feet or hands. The last one either feet or hands, is somewhat of a gray area. Some say it's better to work on the hands first because it's more hygienic than the feet while others say that when it comes to massage and bodywork it should be feet first before the hands because we want to stimulate circulation towards the heart. It will really depend on what services your client would be availing.

Generally a massage comes first before a facial because you do not want a perfectly clean face to touch even a clean massage cradle. The exception to this is when you have booked a particularly aggressive or any painful procedure (e.g. waxing, extractions, diamond peel/microdermabrasion, etc.) and you do not want to finish with a painful session so might as well book the client with an aggressive facial before a massage so the client leaves fully relaxed.

Nails need to go last or they will get ruined. If you smudge your nails right after a manicure, it is actually not the job of the spa to fix the smudge. But, some spas are happy to do so even a day after. The only time it is slightly annoying is when people won't stop texting, playing with their hair or doing something with their hands during a manicure, then of course, they are going to get smudges.

Hot or Cold

Alternating hot and cold treatments with sauna, Turkish bath, hydrotherapy, etc. is reported to increase the levels of beta-endorphins, the endogenous pain killers that are known to produce a sense of well-being. It's advisable to speak to your doctor first before undergoing these treatments.

Drinking warm water or organic tea like ginger, lemon grass before and after the therapy is encouraged to avoid dehydration.

Awkward Situations

Do not be surprised if you happen to doze off, burp, pass gas, have tummy gurgles or

even (unintentional) physiological erections. They will soon pass so do not get embarrassed as this shows our humanity.

The body can have a lot of responses to therapies offered in the spa especially massage and bodywork. While avoiding food at least one hour before your massage will help, there's still the chance that the client will have tummy gurgles, burp or even pass gas. It's okay, because the body relaxes and the systems get detoxified, thus the body can play all kinds of tricks. Your therapist has seen it all, yet sees you well beyond the call of nature and similar kinds of issues.

For men, there is even a rare possibility that massage will even cause a physiological erection. Therapists do not take this personally as this is a common response to nervous system activation. In order to treat the situation accordingly and redirect your attention, ask the therapist to alter the pressure or move to a different area of the body. Sometimes this means that they have to go to the toilet and are holding it.

Wake Up Time

The spa is a very conducive place to sleep, but other clients may be using the room soon and therapists must be prepared for them. While you are allowed at least 5-7 minutes to ready yourself, please do not take too long. Carefully sit up and allow your body to have enough time
to readjust. If you go too fast, you will feel dizzy. Be careful not to slip when getting off the
massage table, especially if your therapist used oil on your feet.

When your therapist says "your session is over, please take your time getting up". What they are actually saying is "Take your time getting up, but please do not take a nap."

After A Facial

Expect to have a turban around your hair and have it a little messed up after the facial. Therefore it is important to bring your own hair brush/comb or choose a spa that has some form of touch-up station or a hair dresser on staff. You are free to use the dryers and hair products available in these touch-up stations.

If and only if you have strong musical preferences, then the best thing to do is to bring an iPod. But this will not be allowed if you are getting a treatment that works around the face and neck because oils and creams can drip into them. I am also discouraging clients to bring in any gadget at all so as to enjoy the tranquility of the setting and get your money's worth. Remember, the spa is not liable for lost or stolen items left unattended.

Tips, Gratuities and Gifts

Tips are often referred to as an acronym for "to insure prompt service". You might

wonder, "Am I supposed to tip the woman who gave me a tea or who showed me to the dressing room?" When it comes to gratuities, I would personally recommend that a client give generously within their means based on each person's assessment of the service given. Being generous is solely dependent on the giver. A 200 pesos tip for one person might be generous enough for some but not for others. It is ultimately a client's decision whether to tip or not. It is worthwhile to note that many therapists/practitioners who work in spas, massage clinics, and wellness centers especially in Asian countries like the Philippines, earn only a small salary (sometimes as low as 50 pesos a day or approximately a dollar a day) or small fraction or percentage of what you are paying for. So, for them tips are an important part of their income. Therapists really appreciate it if you tip them in cash because if you tip them via credit card, they will not be able to get the money until the end of the payroll cycle.

The tipping norm for spa, massage and bodywork services is similar as you would use in a restaurant, the practitioner/technician who worked on you should get between 15-20% of the full price of the service. An exemption to this are those massages performed in a medical environment where tips are usually not accepted.

As for incidentals, use your judgment. Nobody expects you to tip the person who brings you water. If you feel someone has gone above and beyond their call of duty, if she/he orders a special tea or your lunch, for example, it's certainly nice to give the person an additional monetary reward.

Tips are generally left at the reception desk, which have gratuity envelopes and they are responsible for passing them along to the therapist. Sometimes, gratuity envelopes are given to the client by the therapists themselves.

If you are receiving several treatments with several staff members, leave a separate tip for each one. At a medical spa, you tip the Esthetician or facial therapist, not the medical doctor.

When using a gift certificate, do not assume that a tip is included. Some spas don't allow you to put a tip on the gift card, so if it's not clear ask the front desk.

On rare occasion when the spa owner is the one giving you a massage or giving you a facial, tipping is optional. You don't have to tip the owner. Sometimes they charge more for people who are seniors in their line-up, so they make up for it. In my experience being a spa director, I still accept tips from clients but it will not go to me. I always give it to the concierge/reception area and instruct them to distribute it evenly to all the staff on-duty or it will be used to buy staff lunch or merienda (snacks).

You might think tipping is everything but a quick personal note when you leave your money in an envelope also really makes a difference. Most of the time, a tip envelope or gratuity envelope is provided. Some spas include gratuity in the price, so it's always best to check before tipping.

Spa staffs never expect gifts from clients, but if you are a regular, it's completely appropriate to show some extra love around the holidays or any special occasion. Thank you cards, chocolates for the owner and the staff, flowers, gift certificates or additional cash tips are okay. It's really a good practice to give.

If you are unsure what to do, ask if tipping is customary and what is the policy because some spas also include tips in their service price. Be sure to get clarification on fees and services at the time of booking/scheduling.

Buying Retail Products

You are not in any way obliged to buy anything. If you like their products and want to use them at home, then after the facial or any of your spa sessions, you can always ask if there are products that they sell. Surely, they will introduce you to an array of spa retail products.

Sometimes product retailers offer commission and incentives when someone buys their products, so they tend to hard sell clients. If you are not keen on buying, which you can feel during your conversation, then they should not push too much to the point of annoying you. Just say no! Otherwise, if they do not have products that will suite your lifestyle or skin, then they should not offer anything at all.

Gender Issues

Do you mind if you have a male or female therapist? As a client, it's really up to you. Spas, massage clinics and wellness centers, like any business entities will make every effort to accommodate a guest wishes in this regard. Just bear in mind that during peak times, your request may not be accommodated because of the availability of the staff. Some spas have regulations regarding gender, they may opt-in for same gender only specially if you are in Saudi Arabia or a Middle Eastern country. Authentic Ayurvedic treatments in India are traditionally administered by the same gender for energetic reasons.

Children and Pets

Most spas don't allow children under 16, mainly because they are trying to maintain a calm and relaxing atmosphere for adults. But there is also a growing population of children, pre-teens and teens. Therefore some spas tend to offer treatments based on their requirements. In an adult spa which allows teens and children under 16 years old, they are usually accompanied by an adult or either parent during their treatments. To be sure, check the spa policy in advance. There are also spas that specialize in kids spa services like Little Lamb's Spa in Quezon City.

Comment Cards

The comment cards are valuable information and are a way of saying thank you, other than the gratuity given to the therapist or spa staff. A therapist would like to know how well they provided their service to you, especially if it was great!

Cancellations

Rainy weather, traffic, etc. makes it easier for clients to cancel the appointment. Most practitioners and spa establishments require at least a 24-hour notice to avoid cancellation fees. Short-notice cancellations will generally incur a charge, especially if you have left your credit card number during booking. If you did not come and give prior notice, the practitioner or spa, massage clinic or wellness center has the right to forfeit the paid amount or re-schedule if they are generous, but again, it is their prerogative. On the other hand, spas understand that at times canceling is unavoidable, so give them as much time in advance to cancel your booking if your plans change. Every situation is different, so if you are not sure, check with your therapist or spa about their specific cancellation policies, then honor it.

If you are ill and do not feel well, just stay home. If you have a rash or an athlete's foot, then make sure that it's already healed before going to the spa. Spas have the prerogative of turning away clients with a skin infection in order to protect their therapists.

Promotions

Scout for spa sales, off-season discounts and group buying discounts. Spas love gift certificates or cash certificates because most often than not clients end up spending more money than what's on the gift voucher. So, if you're on a budget decide ahead of time how much you want to spend to make up the difference. Bring extra cash so you can tip your therapist and add more services. Gift certificates, gift checks, or gift cards are generally not convertible to cash. But if you will not use them, then you might as well give it to a friend, sell it at 60 to 70% off or trade it with someone who might be able to use it. Most spas offer special deals, loyalty programs, referral programs, point systems, etc. Make sure you get the most out of your money and enjoy it!

Chapter VI

Fun Behind the Scenes

Ok, so what is so fun or glamorous behind the scenes of a beauty professional, massage therapist or spa therapist? Are these the things you really want to know? Some things are funny and some are disgusting. But this is the reality of our spa industry on what happens and what we do to keep you happy. I shall talk about a few and let you decide on the humor if any.

Before you arrive at the salon or spa, the staff has to prepare for your visit. Sometimes we arrive on time and sometimes the staff is late causing other employees or mangers to get mad at them. Sorry at times employees indirectly take their frustrations out on you the client. Oh yes, the staff complains too just like you, as employees personal problems go to work with them too at times. Hum… we are human.. But, again everyone has to maintain that cute smile and courtesy toward you so he/she can get your big tip even when you show up late!

Product usage mishaps are another thing you might not want to know about. Yes we have a lot of newbies, young professionals, and turnover in this business. Our industry suffers from inefficient training in techniques and product knowledge. We use new products on you all the time and thanks for being our test market! That is how we all learn you know. But, does that esthetician, massage therapist or hairstylist really know what product is best for you? If they are not a seasoned professional or not have kept up on training, or are seeing you for the first time, then they might use the wrong product. The truth is this, not only do spas and salons change brands because of costs, but the product companies keep changing their line. Just go to a cosmetics counter and you will realize that it's almost impossible to keep up what is new. So, please bear with us we just cannot know it all even though you think we do.

Spa Technicians and Massage Therapists may have a lot of set up to do before your arrival. Just like Estheticians, they may have to warm up towels and water, heat wax, soak herbs, prepare wraps, mix or warm up products or oils, heat stones, prepare a bath, and set up special equipment, etc. We enjoy doing this for you but it takes our time and we have to pay attention otherwise we can make mistakes or be unprepared.

Cleaning is another item that is constantly haunting us. I know we should clean as we go, but you know how boring it is! Or how toxic (it means busy) it is on weekends. There is a lot of time involved in set up and take down. Everything must be cleaned and sanitized! This includes your massage table or beauty chair, implements and supplies used, towels, sheets etc. Yea right.. sorry, we try.. time is our biggest factor, and if we or our clients go over on treatment time then these items may suffer.! I do apologize that sometimes our sheets or towels are not always washed and disinfected after each session. I do not know of many clean freaks in our industry. But of course, we try to make everything as impeccably clean as we can.

So, I shall list some funny things that humor us as Industry Professionals. Pardon us for being amused. No pun intended but these instances happen:

1. The therapist fails to lock their door to the massage room and another client walks in.

2. The client fails to lock their door and the therapist fails to knock first then seeing the client naked.

3. The client goes into the wrong room and has the wrong treatment done on them.

4. The therapist goes into the wrong room and halfway through the massage or facial discovers that she is working on the wrong client.

5. A male client has a Brazilian wax and tries to wear the spa thong made for women.

6. A spa couple gets caught making out in the sauna, hot tub, or bathroom.

7. The client is showering in the wrong room when the opposite sex comes in.

8. A client falls asleep snoring on the massage table and the therapist cannot wake them up.

9. A client farts while the therapist is working on them.

10. The wrong couple gets a treatment that they did not ask for.

11. The client walks away from the spa forgetting to pay.

12. A client sneezes while having a facial mask on.

13. A client walks out of the facial room to go to the bathroom with the facial mask on.

14. The couple is split up and then brought together as a different couple.

15. A client gives the wrong tip to a therapist that did not work on them. (the massage room was dim you know!)

16. A family has treatments done and the wrong family members are nude together.

17. A client is having a body wrap with bandages and wearing a sauna suit. They ask if they can walk around, the spa therapist says yes, so they go outside of the spa on the street.

18. Clients have to smoke, so they go out the side door and get locked out having to go around the building back through the front entrance with their towel or robe on.

19. This happens to most newbie clients because they do not understand. They are told to get undressed and lie down on

the massage table. The therapist comes in to the room and they are naked on top of the sheet or towel.

20. A client goes inside the solarium and gets a tan only to find out that they misadjusted the machine and they got too tanned or burned. They walk away feeling like they've been barbecued.

Fun behind the scenes is not always so fun for you and yes there are nightmares for us. There are those times when things go very bad.

Like when the new hairstylist might burn your scalp while doing color or waxing and cutting you with the scissors or clippers. The Nail technician hurts your nails while pulling off your fake nails, or burns your skin with the acetone, or burns your feet in the hot water of the foot bath. The Esthetician rips your hair off taking part of the skin causing a scar or the Brazilian waxing gets ugly because you are sweating and in pain, or they burn your face by keeping the glycolic peel on too long. The Spa Therapist leaves the scrub on too long and it half dyes your skin or not all the mud will come off your body from being left on too long, or the sea salt burns your skin because of home shaving. Lastly, the Massage Therapist has gone way too deep and you have visible bruises or a stiff neck the next day, or the hot stones have burned you. Sorry about all these and in behalf of the all the brouhaha behind the scenes we do apologize in advance, staffs including myself are human and do make mistakes. And no I did not commit those mistakes just in case you were wondering. These are compilations of observations, both personal and professional experiences, stories from others I have heard of, etc.

Please be patient because everyone inside the spa, massage center or wellness center really wants to make you feel better about yourself! We want what is best for you and everyone is trying their best to change for the better and improve service.

Chapter VII

Mars in the Planet of Venus

Are men really from Mars and women from another
planet??

When it comes to wants and needs, maybe so. After all,
each one of us is created differently by God for a purpose. But
what about being physical when it becomes very personal (non-
sexual) touch? Do men like to be touched for the attention by
either sex or because they never could get enough of it as a child.
Maybe their parents never used physical touch with them. Why do
some people like to be touched and some do not? Well the debate
can go on and on. So I do not want to dwell on it.

Let me list the top ten things both women and men should
know about the Spa Industry from a male therapist's point of view
from knowing and working with many male therapists thru the
years.

1. A true professional does not care if you are male or female.
    He is concerned about you having a comfortable, relaxing,

and enjoyable experience. So be on time and tell the therapist what you want, remembering that we are not bone poppers (Chiropractors).

2. I am not staring at your body when I am working on you as I am thinking about your body needs and responses to my treatments. I do not care about your body shape, size, or anatomy (yes I have seen it all), and if you shaved your legs or not. Let me leave the room before you undress.

3. Personal hygiene is very important as well as your attitude toward me. Please take a shower, use deodorant, take a breath mint, and treat me with respect. Do not grab me on the table!

4. If you want me to use oils on you then you have to take your undergarments off. Do not worry I will professionally drape you.

5. We drape because we are professionals. No I will not massage you in the nude or give happy endings….yes women like them too! Do not play with your anatomy or grind the table.

6. I will not discuss or embarrass you should you happen to have an accidental orgasm or emission because of the pleasure.

7. I will not embarrass you if your emotions run wild on the table and they are expressed. Some people weep, cry, or sigh.

8. Some people even snore, I don't mind, it just means I am doing my job relaxing you to the point of giving you a must needed sleep.

9. Tell me if you have to go to the toilet, need a tissue, need the music's volume adjusted higher or lower, are too hot or cold, need deeper or lighter pressure, want the lights adjusted, need water or tea, want a breath mint, etc. If you have to belch or fart, give me some warning if I am working on those areas. Remember I cannot read your mind.

10. Turn off your cell phone. You disrupt the energy flow in the room and it takes away your treatment time. You may talk with me briefly during our session or tell me if you

want me to be quiet. What you do share with me in our session is confidential and will not be shared, even if I have your friends or family as clients.

Ok, one more thing... I want your repeat business if you are kind and tip well! (This is service and I work for tips.) Yes, next time I will be more inclined to give you extra time or an extra free service.

Why do men have a beauty, spa or facial treatment? Here is a list of five possible reasons:

1. We come for touch and relaxation. Pampering is wonderful! If women can have this pleasure then we, men want it too! Sadly some of us just use massage for sex or a happy ending, but that is another unprofessional area that we will leave alone.

2. It's important esthetically also for our image to look top notch. Hair perfect, mustache or beard shaped, hand and toe nails trimmed, skin exfoliated, shaven, body hair trimmed, hair dyed, face smooth and unblemished, etc.

3. We might have been pampered as a child and enjoy the different senses and smells, or the complete opposite is that they have never been touched. This may be the only touch some men receive from others.

4. We would like someone to talk to about our personal physical or emotional problems. Humm….. Sometimes a beauty professional listens more than spouses or a girlfriend. Men and women really do confide in their beauty professionals.

5. Special occasions, friends or family do it. Wife or friend drags me along and I am curious.

Why do males go for female massage therapists other than sex? Seven possible reasons:

1. They do not want deep pressure or they think the woman cannot hurt them.

2. They want to be in control of the massage session and can be very picky.

3. If they go to a male, then he must be gay. Phobia about being touched by a male. If they tell their friends, then they might think they are bi-or gay too.

4. It may be the only female touch they get... aloneness.

5. If they have a great body, their hope is to get a compliment or even a date. (Yes, this happens a lot!) Female therapists are humans too!

6. Their wife will not let them go to a male, so both go together at the same time to only females.

7. They can talk with them about their female relationship problems. The therapist will listen and give her input.

Why do men go to men massage therapists other than gay sex? Seven possible reasons:

1. They like strong deep pressure.

2. They can be themselves and will not be judged by their erection or the size of it.

3. Their wife will not let them go to a female due to trust issues.

4. They can have male bonding time about wife/girlfriend problems, sports or politics.

5. This is the only therapist available at that time.

6. Their culture dictates it.

7. They are not as shy when asking for what they need worked on their body.

Overall, there are so many reasons why men go to women or men. We have just scratched the surface and are not debating it, just trying to get a brief understanding. Also, there are so many reasons why women go to women or women go to men, but what is important is that just like love, the human body desires to be touched in a loving way. There are so many reasons why we do what we do. Touch is longed for from infancy. Studies have shown that babies who get touched often and lovingly live a happier healthy life.

As a Martian in the world of Venus, it is as enjoyable as being in our own world.

DISCLAIMER

This publication is designed to inform and educate the public regarding the subject matter covered. The authors have taken reasonable precautions in the preparation of this book and believe the facts and data presented in the book are accurate as of the date it was written. However, neither the author nor the publisher assumes any responsibility for any errors or omissions. The author and publisher specifically disclaim any liability resulting from the reading or application of the information contained in this book, and the information is not intended to serve as a legal advice related to individual situations.

ACKNOWLEDGMENT

All glory to Jesus Christ our Lord and Savior who has inspired us to write this book.